WHY YOGA WORKS

THE SCIENCE BEHIND THE YOGA

Why YOGA WORKS

The Science Behind the Yoga

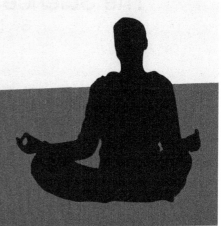

BY MORGAN LEE

Why YOGA WORKS
The Science Behind the Yoga
By: Morgan Lee

Why YOGA WORKS The Science Behind the Yoga, By Morgan Lee

www.ashtanganurse.com

Contents:

WHO IS THE TEACHER?

I was going through my resume the other day and I noticed that I had listed "ability to multi-task" as a skill. I recall writing that on my first resume years ago when I applied to work at a bookstore. It sounded professional and positive, like I could get things done. I kept copying it onto one resume after the other and onto the one after that. However, I have now deleted it from my current resume. I DO NOT multi-task. I focus on one job and get it done quickly and efficiently with successful results. Only then do I move on to the next task but with the same focus, drive, and determination to see it through.

All throughout my childhood I was told to focus. Focus on homework, reading, cutting the vegetables, focus on the teacher. Yet no one ever taught me how to focus. They teach reading, numbers, PE, art, and just about everything else, but they don't teach kids how to focus, how to direct the mind.

I remember in 1992 I wanted a Sony portable CD player, the Discman. I had seen them advertised in the Sunday newspaper and had even held one at Circuit City in Coconut Grove, FL. I was fascinated by the flashy yellow and the grey seal thing that the Walkman had that made it water resistant. This was their top of the line Anti-Shock portable awesomeness. I remembering thinking that if I had that, I would be set for those long family road trips we used to take. I could listen to music instead of pushing my sister into a corner of the car and then getting yelled at for not playing nicely with her. I could be in my own little world. The only problem was that it cost $200.

I made $20 every two weeks for mowing the lawn, so the math didn't quite work in my favor.
I had a goal in mind though. Work for five months and then buy this thing that would make me cool (maybe only "cool" to my sister, because let's be real, I was a dork). Except, there were all these things that got in the way. A CD alone was about $20 and Metallica, Pearl

Jam, Nine Inch Nails, and Nirvana had these kick ass albums that I listened to at my friends' houses which I knew would be good for my trips. I could save for six months and get at least a CD and the Discman. However, going to the movies, video games, comic books, were all things that ate into capital from my Discman fund. Plus, what good is a Discman if I don't have any CD's to listen to...So, naturally, five months turned into seven, and then 10, and that summer family road trip where I was supposed to be listening to music on my portable Discman ended up being a gospel caravan, in praise of Jesus and Margaret Thatcher's biography on tape. If only I had focused. . .

Cut to being 18 applying for a corporate bookstore job where they asked the infamous question, "Can you multi-task?"
"Sure!" And it was true! I can't focus on a damn thing. I'm great at multi-tasking.

I'm 18, I can drive stick shift, hold a cup of coffee, smoke a cigarette, and make a left-hand turn, all at the same time. I got really good at "multi-tasking" on the job too. I could help a customer find a book, answer the phone, ring up another customer, and hit on my co-worker all at the same time.

Working as a nurse was the ultimate test of my multi-tasking prowess. There is no end to what a nurse can get done at the same time with six patients, three doctors, two discharges, one illegible order, and a bladder that hadn't been emptied in ten hours. What helped me to get through it all, though, was having goals. They were distant points on the horizon that I was aiming for.

When I was running, I set clear goals. First, it was to quit smoking and run a 5k. Then a 10k, a half-marathon, then run a faster 5k, a faster 10k, a marathon. Then run longer. I had to set time aside for these runs. Make time for the training runs. I had to eat clean foods before my interval training and time my water breaks on long runs. Sometimes there were setbacks, a rolled ankle, knee pain, a shin splint, a broken hand, but the goal was clear cut. I knew that the short-term fun of Friday night drinking and eating pizza would cripple my Saturday AM run. I stuck to my plan, to the goal. I checked off every goal I had running.

Yoga, however, was a bit fuzzier for me. I didn't have a goal in mind when I started. I didn't have a plan. I was taking Vinyasa flow classes to stretch and complement my running. The Ashtanga Yoga Practice, the method, the sequence, this was all goal oriented and made sense to me. At the time, I believed that in order to progress I had to unlock the previous asana. I looked at how I could get further, what was the next asana? What asana came before in the sequence that could help me with that particular challenge. It was Newton's 3rd Law, for every action there is an equal and opposite reaction, happening every day right in front of me. To be more accurate, it was happening inside of me.

When I discovered Ashtanga Yoga I was still multi-tasking. I was riding 10 miles a day on a bike, running 20 miles a week, stretching in yoga classes, and drinking and eating whatever and whenever I wanted. I worked as a medical assistant and went to college for nursing. I was all over the place, and it was fun... until it wasn't.

The layers of our mind can be pulled back and exposed in practicing Yoga, because we come face to face with our spiritual journey every morning. Through a system of patterns and repetition, the body is trained. The mind, breath, nervous system, digestive system, and circulatory system are trained, focused, and purified. The structure of a yoga practice allows the student to gain control over their mind and the environment they're creating. It gets "easier" for the memory cells to repeat their patterns because of the frequency of the structure that are repeated. When the layers are being pulled apart and exposed, that is when the real work is being done. Those are the moments when the teacher is holding the space safe, allowing the student's mind to train itself, gain control, and grow.

Each of us who enters the the yoga room to practice has a something we're dealing with.

As a teacher I have had the honor of working with clients recovering from gunshot wounds, strokes, PTSD, scoliosis, fractures, pregnancy, fibromyalgia and the list goes on. I've held the space for them to work through their layers, to find love and trust within themselves. The exposure and revelation behind each layer affects not only our individual selves, but everyone we interact with.

Each of us is healing.

NONE OF US ARE OUR INJURY OR DISEASE!

It is our duty to keep the body in good health, otherwise we'll be unable to keep the mind strong and focused.

There is this monkey running around inside our heads, narrating our story, giving us opinions, whining, squealing with joy, and mostly, just confusing the hell out of us. That monkey doesn't want to sit in a class where it will learn to shut up and go away. So that monkey talks, loudly.
What's your excuse today, monkey?

At any time of day there are things that are more fun, more exciting, less painful, and more lucrative than doing yoga. There are a million excuses that you can come up so that something more fun seems like a better alternative to focusing on the Self. But how many times have you screamed at that monkey to shut up!? Has it ever worked?

How many times has the monkey been wrong?

Letting the monkey control this thing called "you", is like giving the monkey keys to your brand new Tesla. It's probably going to bite them, throw them, and take a crap on it; unless you train the monkey how to handle the keys.

That is precisely what yoga is doing: training the monkey. Focusing.

CAN YOGA ASANA BENEFITS BE EXPLAINED SCIENTIFICALLY?

The first book about yoga that I bought was The Yoga Mala, by K. Pattabhi Jois. It is his treatise regarding the yoga asana in the Primary Series of the Ashtanga Yoga Method. It is the main point of reference for the physical practice of the primary series, as well as a prescription for curing ailments.

I wrote much of it off as pure bologna. I wasn't persuaded by claims that an asana could purify the ribs (whatever that means) cure constipation and hemorrhoids, and a bunch of other things that went against my western medical training. I didn't understand The Yoga Mala and what Jois was getting at in his book: ten asanas remove "bad fat" from the stomach, ten asanas purify the anal canal, while others increase digestive fire, purify the kidneys, etc. It was rubbish.

The entire book seems to me at the time, focused on clearing the digestive system. In fact, it's with a bit of shame that it has taken me a while to understand what was being laid out before me. I was reading the book thinking that each asana is like an individual pill. That Ardha Baddha Padmottasana was the equivalent to Gas-X, an anti-flatulence pill; because the benefits listed were "quells the gas that arises from inappropriate food" and "prevents gas from occurring in the stomach." What I failed to understand was that the asana, the yoga shape, is like a single herb in a formula. The formula IS the yoga practice.

A formula is like a soup. It's made up of many herbs, and spices, with each herb having a specific dose, an amount to be included in the formula, and an order in which each ingredient is added. Forgetting one ingredient, or adding too much of another, throws the entire soup off balance and ruins it.

When cooking, one must sauté the onions before sautéing the garlic. If you do the garlic first, it will burn and make the soup bitter. You can also think of the yoga sequence as putting on your shoes before your pants. It can be done, but you will dirty the inside of your pants, perhaps tear them, and you will certainly struggle with getting your ankles through. So following a sequence is indeed important. It is why a student should follow the particular vinyasa - the inhale and exhale, the meditation, and the focus on muscle contractions. Otherwise we are simply doing exercises.

Exercise in this way is like eating food because we are hungry and not thinking about food as medicine. On its own, the individual asana helps to resolve a particular function, but it is the unique pattern and frequency in the formula that cures and makes us aware of our true Self.

PRACTICING BEYOND

I'm doing a terrible thing and assuming you're practicing yoga for more than just exercise. A yoga practice works to improve the body, mind, and soul. If the students simply focus on improving the mind, no amount of intellect will save you from a heart attack. Equally so, focusing only on the soul will create a union with the Devine, but the body and mind will suffer a short existence that does not improve the general welfare of society. If you are doing a yoga practice for exercise, then the body will look and function but you will be trapped in the most superficial planes of existence.

Yoga works to unite the three beings of what makes you unique.

Let's say that you have some unresolved emotions. Who doesn't? Rather than dealing with these emotions that make you hot and bitter every time you talk about them or deal with that situation, you stuff it. You box it up and place it on a shelf inside the wall of protection you have been building since childhood. This wall is made up of similar boxes. Conflicts that are unresolved which may have frightened the four-year-old child inside, but now are a habit for the adult you.

The four-year-old didn't have the skills or tools to deal with the issues at the time, but adult you choose to close the lid and look away. Adult you seals it inside the wall with alcohol, drugs, sweets, etc. Whatever it takes to take the bitter taste from your mouth. You drink a Frappuccino. It's cool, it's sweet, the creamy smooth liquid pacifies your unresolved emotions.

It tastes good. It's a resolution. No more heat, no more bitterness. Eventually, one Frappuccino turns into six. The excessive sugar is metabolized as "storage" and is eventually deposited into the uterus or prostate.

If you are practicing Yoga for exercise and ignoring the idea of it being a formula to unite the body, mind, and soul, the practice may be a means of escape, a Frappuccino. Something that we 'do' to escape the very reality that we are boxing up.

Through practicing the correct physical asana and breathing techniques, diseases will be cured, BUT, there is of course, an exception. There is always an exception. In this case, if we keep eating foods that drive our unresolved emotions deeper inside us, it can actually lead to an increase in sickness.

Looking at Marichyasana A,B,C & D as a progressive sequence, since I spent a good bit of time there when learning the Primary Series. These guys restore the digestive power, eliminating flatulence, indigestion, and constipation. In women, the womb becomes strong. The asana themselves place pressure on certain points that aid digestion according to Traditional Oriental Medicen. Points that help the large and small intestines, the pancreas, the stomach, liver, and the kidneys. Preforming the asana alone and eating foods that do not promote health will not restore digestive fire. That is Einstein's definition of insanity.

The asana is a reminder that we are probably eating too fast, not chewing our food enough, or eating too much sugar, since that is the number one cause of flatulence.

Gas is a natural product of bacterial fermentation in the large intestine. Excess flatulence is often a result of eating beans, brussels sprouts, cabbage, bread, sugar, beer, and dairy products. If we slow down when eating, chew our food properly, and eliminate foods causing these digestive issues, then we have mastered the point of asana. "Getting the bind" is the result of doing these things, but it is not indicative of the correct understanding of the asana. If we cannot get the bind in Mari D, should we move on to the next asana?

The next asana, Navasana, also increases digestive fire, and in terms of health and practicing to resolve digestive issues; this is the last asana that aids digestion. Medically speaking, I see no issue practicing Navasana to help restore one's digestive fire. The full practice to that point is about an hour long and if the student has not taken any food since going to sleep, that is about 12 hours of fasting*, and enough time to kick into gear the gastric juices that begin digesting food correctly.

In the greater hierarchy of needs, digestion comes before reproduction, and one should have a healthy digestive system to ensure a long life, a life that can care for their offspring.

A yoga practice is designed to heal and restore the basic needs of an individual before working on their psychological needs; the needs involving intimate relationships, family, friends, achievement, and respect. Those all come only if we have a sense of safety and proper nutrition/digestion.

* Eight hours of sleep, last meal two hours before sleep, awake 30 minutes before practice, one hour practice, 30 minutes after practice waiting to eat; 12 hours.

PRIMITIVE NATURE

I wanted to talk about the digestive system, but I can't talk about digestion without first taking a side road into pain and the "fight or flight" mechanism, as they are related. All organ systems are interconnected and dependent on each other. Together they make up the whole that we are as we go along on our spiritual journey.

If we practice a yoga sequence in a specific order like a formula, then it is a medicine taken to heal. It is important to look at how a yoga practice first heals our basic human needs.

The first most basic human need is to move away from pain and suffering. In a limited sense, this is just showing up every day, standing on the mat. *Ekam, inhale lifting the arms up*. Period. Simply showing up to class in the morning is moving away from the pain and suffering of our life before we practice.

Prior to all this yoga business, I was inauthentic. I played the game of life. It was my own version of hell. If things didn't go my way, if I didn't win, then it was the world's fault. Society was to blame for me not having enough money to live on. The world was out to get me. Women were manipulative and men were terrible. I could go on about blaming everyone else for my problems, but you already understand this pain.

Sometime after running and into this yoga thing, I began to understand that I was responsible for my actions or my inactions. If I wasn't making enough money at my job and there was no room for growth, it was time for a revolution. It was time for massive change. The world isn't out to get me, women aren't manipulative. I didn't know what I wanted and I was allowing myself to be swayed. I needed to take responsibility for my actions. Taking responsibility for your actions is being authentic.

When I started practicing, I really began taking action to move away from pain. *Dve, exhale.*

An organism, EVERY ORGANISM, must move out of pain before it can work on other physiological needs. Then it can focus on digestion and eventually reproduction. Plants, humans, animals, and even bacteria, must move away from pain before focusing on the finer qualities of living.

We are fragile beings and by some miracle, we make it into adulthood. As living, breathing, humans, we continually teeter between chaos and order. The foods that we eat, the air that we breathe, send parts of our body's ecosystem into an acidic state, chaos. The body offsets this with a specific order, removing calcium from the bones to balance the acid, exhaling CO_2, etc. The body balances itself between these two states, walking a thin line. Too much chaos or order sends the body into disaster.

In order to balance the body, we have a highly developed nervous system. It balances chaos and order. It is divided into two sections. The section responsible for order functions automatically, it's on auto-auto-pilot. We call this the autonomic nervous system. No cognitive thought goes into making this system work (not much cognitive thought went into naming it either). It is a brilliant, simple system that takes care of the necessary functions of life and living.

The autonomic nervous system is our internal locus of control. It is responsible for organ function; heart rate, respiratory rate, digestion, the pupil's response to light, urination. Basic coughing, sneezing, swallowing, or vomiting are also possible because of the autonomic nervous system.

Because scientists can't leave good enough alone, or there needs to be a yang for every yin, they divided this autonomic system into two components that work opposite each other. One component takes care of "feeding and breeding" and its antagonist, the "fight or flight" mechanism.

The "fight or flight" system is called the sympathetic nervous system. It's quick to respond, as it stems from the most primitive part of the brain, the part associated with self-preservation. It's like when you stand up from sitting, the sympathetic system jumps into action to prevent a sudden loss of blood to the head by regulating heart rate and blood pressure. The primary muscle we often associate with "fight or flight" is the psoas muscle. This is the muscle that burns when we hold the leg out in utthita hasta padangusthasana in the 7th and 14th vinyasa. The psoas' instinctive nature is to help us get away quickly. It's why that muscle burns when the count is slow.

When we perceive danger via visual or physical stimuli, the brain sends a signal to the adrenal glands. The message is simple: kill or be killed. This message is flashed out to the rest of the body saying that we need to take action. Epinephrine is released into the blood stream from the adrenal glands located above each kidney. Epinephrine is a chemical that flies around in the blood shutting down non-essential organs, like in that Star Trek episode where Kirk is demanding Scotty to give us more power, so Scotty re-routes power from one system to boost the thrusters so they get maximum warp. The body responds to this signal by opening up the blood vessels in some areas and closing down other systems. Our heart rate speeds up. We breathe faster to oxygenate the surging blood rushing around our vital organs and muscles. Blood moves away from the organs that deal with digestion. We have a limited amount of time to make use of this response before it burns out and we have either made it or made a meal for someone far bigger than us.

We need these special systems to escape pain, danger, or the threat of pain and danger. It's a mechanism for self-preservation. Order is necessary. It builds structures and society. Without the autonomic system, we would not be here. We would not be able to sleep. Chaos is necessary however, to spur change and innovation. In this case, chaos is what we control. This part of the nervous system is called the somatic nervous system, or the voluntary nervous system. This is the arm reaching for the coffee or the alarm's snooze button. This is the system that gets us into "trouble" by reaching for that extra cookie, and takes us to the moon.

We need one foot in order and the other in chaos. Controlled chaos is the diaphragm contracting and remaining contracted. Remaining while the carbon dioxide builds up in the blood stream and the oxygen is depleted. The mind becomes restless, distracted. We stress out. Eventually we either give in or pass out and the autonomic nervous system kicks in and takes over lung functionality once more.

By slowing down our breathing in stressful situations, we train our brain to focus and remain calm and make rational decisions. With continued practice, we train our body to operate more efficiently. The US Navy Seals go through a training that "is designed to push you mentally to the brink, over and over again, until you are hardened and able to take on any task with confidence, regardless of the odds - or until you break." - The Red Circle, Brandon Webb. Notice any similarities with Yoga?

In our yoga practice, we go to that place of fear every day. Our anxious minds race between thoughts: will I break? Will I have the energy? Did I eat too much last night? Did I have a BM before class? Can I do this and get to work on time? When we train our breathing, we train our heart to slow down because our muscles demand less oxygen. Our lungs can exchange oxygen and carbon dioxide more effectively, and with higher profusion in the alveolar lining. We will learn more about this when we discuss the circulatory system. We become individuals who no longer react to stress, but respond to it. We can become creative individuals because we can control the stress rather than react to it, and because of that, we can evolve our society and our individual being.

If we do not control this stress reaction, it may develop into PTSD and/or numbing via any number of methods. Remember, the body fights to preserve vital organs, the heart, and brain. But, the body cannot sustain functioning in a stressful environment. For one, digestion stops and if we don't get the required nutrients, the body burns itself up.

GOALS & DRUGS

There is a difference between setting goals and being focused. One leads to burnout, the other is a pathway to seeing lifelong progress.

A goal is a result, a future you: one you intend to reach. You may reach it, celebrate for a minute or two, then get up and set a new one. There is never-ending satisfaction. "Anytime you finish a climb, there's always the next thing you can try." - Alex Honnold, *Free Solo*

In yoga there is always another asana. Does this sound familiar? Intermediate series is like a drug. Students line up just to watch other students do Sharath's Led Intermediate class at KPJAYI. They show up before the students who are actually in the class. They show up to watch the back bending, the arm balance, the twisted pretzel legs behind the head. They show up because Intermediate is a fantastic drug. You can only take the drug if you are cool enough to stand up from a back bend. Nobody wants to watch primary.

Dopamine, a naturally occurring organic chemical produced by the body, plays a major role in our "reward-motivated behavior." It places a value on an outcome which motivates an organism to achieve said outcome, the "reward". The yoga practice continues to feed and reward the nervous system. Now that you can stand up, bend further. Now that you can bend further, bend the other way. We get conditioned to want more. It stimulates our pleasure center.

The primary functions of a Catecholamine, the drug class that dopamine belongs to, are to elicit a positive emotion; which effects our decision making and our behavior. The pleasure we feel from the release of dopamine is our reward, and we want that reward. We watch videos on how to: deepen our backbends, open our hips, strengthen our shoulders, balance on our hands in a backbend with our legs behind the head. We watch Led Intermediate. We attend yoga conferences, workshops, confluences, retreats, and festivals. We pay trainers.

Rewarding stimuli is the basis for much of our learning. Think Pavlov and his dogs. Humans and money, or sex. We seek pleasure. It's a natural instinct. We learn from this pleasure. We learn to associate certain things with this pleasure/reward. It is learned from childhood and we continue to develop it throughout our lives. It is a basic biological trait. From the simplest protozoa to bacteria and complex organisms, such as humans, we are attracted to things that stimulate this pleasure center. For the most part, we are attracted to sweets and repulsed by bitter or sour flavors. We learn to understand what is sweet, like a bar of chocolate, and we want to eat that chocolate because we know that the reward is delightful. When we have sweets, dopamine is released. Eating a bar of chocolate is similar to opening a gift on your birthday, or in the case for yoga, achieving a new pose, assuming that one has found a comfortable seat in the previous asana.

Some of us need that bar of chocolate, that dopamine hit harder than others. Some of us require a higher level of dopamine to be released before feeling like we have received the "reward." It's all relative to the individual. If you need more, it doesn't mean that you are a bad person. It simply means that you require greater stimuli. If we apply that concept to yoga, then it means that you require more poses to be stimulated. I loved the next asana like a fat kid loves cake. I loved that it felt like Christmas when I got a new asana. I had a new gift to unwrap. I had something to play with. For a day, maybe a week, the dopamine ran high. I was excited.

The problem with a drug, or a chemical dependent feeling, is that when the chemical is depleted, so is the feeling. Being dependent on things outside yourself to stimulate pleasure doesn't feel healthy, but I didn't know of any other way to be happy. From an early age, we are given teething tools to ease our discomfort with cutting teeth. As we grow we are given toys to play with, rewarded for grades in school, given raises at our jobs for . . . doing our job. All of these are external factors that stimulate a moment of joy. When the feeling was fresh, I felt like I could sustain this yoga practice forever. When I got a raise I could tolerate the job for another couple of months, it would take maybe only a few weeks before complaining again. When the feeling was fresh it stimulated the reward center and I focused on a goal. I could commit my heart to the job and the people I work with. In my yoga practice it meant becoming proficient in a pose to feel comfortable in it and incorporate it into my daily asana practice. The practice became longer and longer with the rest of the postures that at one time gave me that dopamine rush. Only they no longer gave me the high they once did. They no longer elicited that dopamine response.

How do I get back to that level again? A new pose. How do I get a new pose? Get good at this one, get really good. Do the homework, watch the videos, do extra practice work. Hire a private tutor to give me the "secrets" to working through this asana. Show up every day and show the teacher what I can do. That's how this practice works. A teacher acknowledges where you are and then gives you the next pose, the next dose of dopamine.

With goals we tend to push limits. Because we are living for a future, we get anxious about where we are now. We force things to open before they are ready. I pulled my back and tore my QL muscle because I was addicted to the hit. I know students who have torn their meniscus, who slipped discs in their vertebrae, who become anorexic, all for the pose. The reward from our teacher. The next hit. This is how we OD on yoga. We get burned out.

With a goal there are two scenarios. We reach said goal. We celebrate. We set a new goal. OR we don't reach said goal. We try again. Again. Again. Again. If we depend on a release of dopamine to practice then we are dependent on something outside of ourselves. What happens if we fail again, and again, and again, and we don't receive the reward? Is this the point we face ourselves in the mirror? Is this when the real yoga begins?

Practicing yoga does not guarantee a good life. In fact, I'm not sure what the good life is. I know what a good life isn't. I've listened to some country music and line danced before. There are some pretty good descriptions in those songs about living a lousy life. But I'm not quite certain that I can explain or give a definition of what a good life actually is. I understand that the measure of a good life has to do with a measure of inner-happiness. I can also see how being financially well off and having a measure of exterior success can lead to inner-happiness. Measuring success by having a particular asana practice, a certain number of followers, or a certain amount in a savings account, are all valid measurements of success. They can be scientifically quantified with a particular value. I get it. Yet scientific studies have shown that beyond a particular dollar amount, happiness doesn't increase, and if they were to study yoga asana, I'm sure they would find the exact same conclusion. Beyond a certain asana, the level of happiness doesn't increase as exponentially as one might figure. It may actually take away a level of happiness.

People who are concerned with external success compare themselves to others who have "more" of that success than they do, rather than comparing themselves to those who have less.

For instance, when I was learning the primary series of the Ashtanga Yoga Method, I would often compare myself to other students in the room who were well beyond my skill level at the time. I didn't have the tools that develop with a yoga practice, yet I compared myself to these students. Even worse, was when a new student came along and flew through the series while my (insert negative self-talk here) was stuck at Marichyasana D. I could in fact argue that at a certain point, the Ashtanga Yoga Method actually borders on a level of unhappiness. Sometimes we are unhappy with the commitment; the early mornings, the frequency of practice, the rigidity and structure.

Unhappiness is there and continues to remain present in the practice until the student realizes that they are measuring their happiness on the external, if the student remains with the practice. At what point does the student realize that they must shift their focus towards the internal? I don't have any quantifiable data, and it would be correct to say that this realization happens at different levels throughout the practice. One could say that this "awakening" happens daily. The realization that happiness is determined from within, practiced daily, and refreshed by a yoga practice, IS a pretty good measure of a good life. It doesn't however guarantee a good life. It doesn't guarantee that shitty things won't happen, and that we won't react like a child. It doesn't guarantee a set income, a delayed flight, or a first-class ticket. It simply gives us the tools to handle life. How to handle the delayed flight at an airport without resorting to name calling and berating the customer service representative who had nothing to do with personally delaying YOUR flight. It gives us the tools to be respectful to our parents, siblings, spouse, kids, boss, coworkers, and everyone around us.

EMBRACING THE DARK SIDE: COFFEE

It's one of the world's most widely used drugs. It's an adenosine antagonist, and it's delicious!
I take mine black, single origin (Unblended), in a V60 pour over. I prefer a light roast because of the more complex flavors.

I became addicted to the drug in Mysore, on my first trip to India. In southern India it is typically "diluted" with chicory. Chicory adds a subtle chocolate taste and cuts down on the bitterness of the dark roast. It was originally added to coffee in France when Napoleon placed a tax on the good stuff. Chicory stretched and sometimes replaced coffee all together, #oldworldproblems.

Let's not kid ourselves though. The root of the bitter endive plant is not a substitute for the delicious single-origin brew.

Coffee and the effects of caffeine can improve attention, dilate the bronchial tubes, improve memory, and stimulate bowel movements. Caffeine has been proven to enhance muscle strength and power* and increase the body's metabolism. However, it also elevates your blood pressure by constricting the blood vessels. Caffeine can also enhance the effects of NSAIDs (Motrin), but so can ginger and turmeric.

It doesn't actually get you wired, but coffee works by blocking adenosine receptors, which the body uses to trigger its "sleep mode". With caffeine in place of adenosine in the receptors, the body has no breaks as it cruises down the freeway doing 110 with increasing levels of dopamine, whereas adenosine is quite useful. Adenosine can convert a tachycardic (fast) heart rate if the patient is experiencing SVT's.

Coffee doesn't stimulate the need to urinate. It has no diuretic effect.** If you feel the urge to go to the bathroom during class, something else is tickling your junk. Urination is controlled by at least five areas of the brain,*** possibly more, but scientists have mapped five as of 'now'. That's a lot of Vritti's! In some species urinating is a form of social communication; communicating social rank, and sexual status. Most of us living in a "civilized" society urinate in socially appropriate and environmentally safe areas. One's version of a civilized socially appropriate area to void in, varies by culture. It is not uncommon to see a person on the side of the road using a rice field or bush as an "appropriate" area. If you have traveled between Bangalore airport and Mysore, you are very familiar with this custom.

There are very precise coordinations between neuro receptors in the bladder and the motor patterns that occur before voiding. Generally, the brain is aroused when the bladder is reaching an established level before the maximum threshold and our behavior must be suspended to move to an appropriate space to void. Ultimately, the descending part of the spinal cord controls bladder function. This is why paraplegics have control over "some" urinary function. That doesn't mean that voiding is only controlled by bladder distention.

During a fight-or-flight response, the bladder is relaxed. The bladder is not a vital organ that will help us get away from danger and it will not defend us. Remember that in a fight-or-flight scenario, blood is diverted to muscles to get away or to fight. Sphincter muscles for digestion, urination, and excretion are on lockdown. Nothing gets out, nothing gets in. In our asana practice we place increased pressure on the bladder; from bandhas, abdominal pressure from navasana, and horrible twists like Mari D. This pressure does facilitate an urge to void. They decrease the space of the bladder, making the urine threshold smaller. But, remember that five areas of the hot mess we call a brain are working to control when we actually void this urine. We decide when we will void it by making the actions to move to an area that is socially accepted for this bodily fluid.

When we feel the need to "GO" in the middle of our asana practice, is it the brain getting away from pain? The brain will look for any out, any excuse to avoid discomfort. We dwell on it until it is overwhelming and we excuse ourselves. Assuming we didn't down a 1-liter bottle of water before class and only had a cup of coffee about an hour before... If we empty the bladder before practice, diuresis (the process of healthy kidney function emptying urine into the bladder) shouldn't be substantial enough to place extra pressure on the part of your spinal cord that gives the urge to relieve oneself in the middle of practice. But you know, Supta Kurmasana is easier when we have our bandhas engaged, our bladder empty, and our stomachs pulled in. That and Navasana is a "perfect" time to skip to the bathroom during led class. *Four . . . ffffffffiii . . . Hey, why are you in a hurry?*

*Grgic J, Trexler ET, Lazinica B, Pedisic Z (2018). "Effects of caffeine intake on muscle strength and power: a systematic review and meta-analysis". *Journal of the International Society of Sports Nutrition.* **15**: 11. doi:10.1186/s12970-018-0216-0. PMC 5839013. PMID 29527137.

**https://www.mayoclinic.org/healthy-lifestyle/nutrition-and-healthy-eating/expert-answers/caffeinated-drinks/faq-20057965

*** Anitha Manohar, Andre L Curtis, Stephen A Zderic, and Rita J Valentino "Brainstem network dynamics underlying the encoding of bladder information" eLife 2017;6:e29917 DOI: 10.7554/eLife.29917 https://www.ncbi.nlm.nih.gov/pmc/articles/PMC5714501/

WHAT ARE YOU EATING THAT IS CONTRIBUTING TO YOUR CURRENT HEALTH?

We search for meaning. I'm even searching for it while writing this. We want to blame something outside of ourselves for our current state of 'being.' Something outside of our power. We like to blame a cold for making us sick, but a virus is incomplete. It's not whole. It needs a host. It's completely dependent on a living organism to replicate. Maybe it's a reminder that we need to slow down? Maybe the "cold" virus is reminding us to stop because we are not taking care of ourselves. We are not paying enough attention to ourselves. Success makes us complacent, conceited.

Poor health is responsible for "disrupting the ability of human beings from pursuing their spiritual journey." - Charaka Samhita A.D. 200, the first Indian text on medicine. If we spend time focusing on our health and taking care of our bodies then perhaps we don't create an environment for the virus to replicate? That's not saying that the virus won't do its due diligence and fulfill its purpose to replicate inside of you. You can be assured that as soon as you take a moment off, it's going to wonder right in your direction.

The practice of yoga asana is a formula designed to keep us paying attention. It keeps us on our toes and keeps us able to pursue our spiritual journey. On a physical level one way the practice restores or sustains our health is by keeping our digestive system strong. The digestive system works to serve the other organ systems; cardiovascular/respiratory, neuro, reproductive, endocrine, etc. These other systems work to keep us on our spiritual path. The digestive system is made up of organs, glands, and tissue. Digestion begins before we take the first bite. It begins with a thought. Maybe it's a delicious odor that triggers a cascading reaction in the body? When we are in pain, we do not sense odors. We cannot detect the smell of fresh baked bread, of the floral notes of coffee opening up as the first drops of water hydrate the thirsty beans. After detecting an odor or another trigger, the salivary glands in the mouth begin to secrete a liquid that will help dissolve and break apart whatever you consume. Gastric acids begin to flood the stomach to assist as well. The digestive system is lengthy to explain in detail, but easy to simplify; you put food in your mouth, chew, swallow, and poop it out.

The Charaka Samhita is an Indian composition of texts from the 2nd century C.E. detailing human body theory, disease pathology, and treatment. It is very similar to the Huang Di Nei Jing of Traditional Oriental Medicine dating back to the first century B.C.E. They both detail the importance of diet and medical diagnoses for the prevention and treatment of a given disease in the human body. They detail in length, the anatomy of the body, the diagnosis, and the prognosis based upon sensory input from the doctor and patient. Chapters on ethics, pathology, philosophy, diet, nourishment, tastes of medicines, and responsibility of the Physician, the Nurse, and the Patient are included. The two books provide a solid foundation to care for, treat, and live a life that is in tune with our spiritual path.

DIGESTION

In his book "Origins", Neil DeGrasse Tyson talks about science evolving and the universe expanding. It's a fantastic read. I took away an understanding that what we know today is valid, but that it doesn't always apply in the future. Science changes, it evolves. It is not the totalitarian rule of the medieval Catholic Church. Thank God! (pun intended)

What we know today to be true is true because we cannot disprove it with technology. That is carefully worded and not to be misunderstood as, "truth is what we can prove." There are some things that exist that we cannot prove... yet. Dark matter being one of those things, according to Tyson. This will come up again when we talk about the reproductive system.

We are evolving. We humans, you and I, along with the universe, plants, animals, and the earth. That's "scientifically" proven and agreed upon by most. We are evolving every second, beyond the concept that the human body is born of new cells every seven years, but inclusive of it too. We are evolving with every experience. Our DNA is coding for new and different proteins every second, proteins that build the pathways to tell the story of our lives. Some cells stay with us through our lives, stomach cells are replaced every few days, and bones about every decade.*

It may seem like a far-out concept to think that we are fundamentally and organically different than who we were even a second ago. But when you are learning to tie your shoelaces, every ounce of your six-year-old body is poured into making the bunny ears, crossing them, and pushing the head down the hole. Maybe it didn't actually go like that, but I'm left-handed, which means that I need to complicate matters. Bless my parents for being patient with me as I tried to figure out what they were showing me backwards, to make some sense of the mess.

At six years old the proteins have not been made yet for us to know how to use our fingers in the particular way needed to tie laces. Each time we experience tying our shoelaces, DNA is coding proteins to establish this pathway. In a few years, one was able to complete this task and carry on a conversation simultaneously because the pathway had long since been established.

Each experience changes our DNA, causes us to evolve. The stages that we went through to simply tie our shoelaces developed from the fine motor skills that preceded it. The pincer grasp at 10 months, the use of the noon dominant hand at three to stabilize an object. We build upon the greatness of our current self to get to the next level. We build up, level upon level, by taking in nutrients and processing them. These nutrients become incorporated to form the proteins that make up our hair, eyes, blood, and movements.

The chemical reactions that take place to maintain our evolution and our spiritual journey is called metabolism. You have probably heard this word thrown around when discussing weight loss. Metabolism is more than just weight loss though. It is the sum of the chemical reactions that take place in an organism. The reactions that build up and break down. The chemical reactions that convert food to fuel, the building blocks of life (protein, lipids, nucleic acids), and remove waste. If you are taking in more fuel food than you are breaking down and using, you are in an energy surplus and the body will store that surplus for use in the future. If you are taking in less calories than you are burning up then the body is in a deficit and the body burns the extra storage it had built up.

When people speak of metabolism related to fat loss they are referring to your metabolic rate, the rate at which your body burns calories. Calories are units of energy, so when people talk about calories they are talking about how fast your body uses energy, how much fire you are burning inside. It's referring to how easy it is for your body to break down or build up a complex carbohydrate into a simple sugar, or how much energy it takes for a nucleic acid to become an amino acid, a nucleotide, or a piece of DNA.

We each have a different metabolic rate, affected by the enzymes and flora that live in our digestive system. Affected by our activities of daily living, as well as our emotions. The easiest product for our body to break down is sugar, followed by carbohydrates, fats, and proteins, in that order. Carbohydrates not broken down and used immediately are stored in the body as fat to be used when the body is calorie deficient. Fats are also necessary. Period. Fats are necessary for our sex hormones to activate. Marvin Gaye will not be singing for you unless you have some body fat. Hair growth, menses, libido, and more; all depend in part on having some fat.

*Barbara J. Campbell, MD, https://orthoinfo.aaos.org/en/staying-healthy/bone-health-basics/

DIGESTION 101 DIGESTED IN 3 MINUTES

Digestion begins in the mouth, chewing food and allowing it to mix with saliva helps to break carbohydrates into smaller pieces. This is the only part of digestion that is under our conscious control. The more time we spend meditating on our food and breaking it into smaller and smaller pieces, the more the body will be able to extrapolate more nutrients. Once we swallow the food it is no longer under conscious control. The autonomic nervous system takes over. The digestive system, under automatic control, only operates if the individual is free from pain and feeling safe.

Food swallowed enters the stomach, where it mixes with gastric juices that further dilute and break apart the now completely unrecognizable lunch. This is the primary area that breaks apart proteins into smaller compounds. Food hangs around for about an hour in the stomach and it is emptied after about two. Powerful muscles in the stomach contract, in a wave-like pattern, processing the food in what is called peristalsis. This partly digested food and gastric juices, called chyme, passes from the stomach into the small intestine. Assisting the breakdown of the chyme in the small intestine is bile and lipase.

Bile is mostly water and salt. It is produced by the liver and stored in the gall bladder. When the chyme enters the small intestine from the stomach it sends a signal telling the gall bladder to release the stored liquid. Bile increases the surface area of fats which are broken down by lipase, the juice secreted by the pancreases. If fats are not broken down this way, and absorbed by the small intestine, we run into a bigger issue down the road at the large intestine which is not equipped to handle fats. Bile also colors our stool that lovely shade of brown. The color comes from bilirubin, the corpses of red blood cells that are old and worn out. The spleen severs them in half and sends them to the liver for processing.

The pancreas is responsible for producing lipase. Lipase is the chief of all digestive juices. It controls the entire symphony of destruction from macro molecules to micro ones. It is also responsible for producing insulin when blood sugar is too high. Insulin moves sugar from the blood into the muscles and other tissue to use as energy. Lipase also produces glucagon, a hormone that tells the liver to turn stored sugar into glucose, aka useable energy.

Most of our digestion takes place in the small intestine, our lower brain. When the food particles are reduced enough in size and composition, they are moved through the small intestine and carried away through our blood stream. Inside the twisting and turning folds of the small intestine are these finger-like protrusions called villi, which increase the surface area of the small intestine. The twisting and folding slows down food, to be properly absorbed, so it can release the maximum amount of nutrients. After most of the useable nutrients are absorbed into the bloodstream, the semi solid mass of chyme enters the large intestine where it travels up the right side of the abdomen. Water is reabsorbed as the chyme travels across and down the left side of the large intestine to the colon. In the colon stool ferments and packs together preparing for defecation. This entire process, from chewing to pooping, usually takes about 12 to 50 hours and varies from person to person.

GETTING THE GOODNESS IN

Plants take in sunlight and nutrients from the soil and metabolize it through a process called photosynthesis. Plants grow and expand, taking in more light and nutrients to eventually reproduce, thus making more plants, to take in more sunlight and more nutrients. We take in air and nutrients from the plants and animals that we eat and metabolize it in a process known as the Krebs cycle. Like plants, we are ever expanding and evolving, reproducing, and coding new DNA that will remake the entire body. So it is important to take in beneficial nutrients. Nutrients that will contribute to a positive evolution.

This evolution is different for each person so I'm not going to begin to profess what "beneficial nutrients" are for you specifically. In general, get some sunlight, breathe in some clean air, drink water, eat. Chew your food. Digest the experience.

In 2004, one of my good friends from high school committed suicide when he was 24.
I know that I will never "get over" him or what he chose to do 14 years ago. It was his choice, but that doesn't mean that the hurt isn't still there. There is still a part of me digesting the entire experience, accepting it and its energy, and allowing it to pass through me. I did try to drink away the hurt at one point. I tried to stuff it down… because that's always healthy. I tried running from it. I ended up running from a lot more than the hurt. I ran from a marriage, my friends, my family, and even my health. I ran because I only knew two modes: on/off. I got fast. I ran a 5k in 22 minutes. But I didn't feel like I was getting anywhere. There was always another time, another race, and running in minus temperatures in Chicago is awful. I covered a lot of ground, but I just wasn't getting anywhere.

When I didn't get anywhere running from my friend's suicide, I went into therapy. I had an amazing therapist and I did a lot of work. There was a lot of breaking down and breaking through to understand that this is an event that has shaped and continues to shape me. Emotions can be painful things to deal with. Most of the time we run away from them. We cover them up rather than confront them. Rather than looking the emotion in the eye and going through it, we allow it to pass through us.

The same goes for all of the nutrients we take in from what we eat. Will you take in what you need and allow the indigestible contents to pass through or will you hold onto them?

BRINGING IT BACK TO THE MAT

We call the small intestine the second brain, but it's actually the first. The enteric nervous system (ENS) present in the abdomen operates independently of the central nervous system (CNS), and it is formed in utero before the CNS.*

We experience emotions through our gut. Along with food, this is where we digest our human experience. All of what we eat is being processed by the body. ALL of what we eat is contributing to our evolution. It's going to take more than a 30-day detox to clean out thousands of DNA-coding proteins. Yet, sometimes all it takes is a second to release a samskara that we have been holding on to, processing. The first time I was invited to Led Intermediate, I spent the hour before practice, anxiously waiting on the steps of the shala. Every "chakrasana, go back" brought me closer to this impending doom I had building up in my head. The two hours before practice had me visiting the toilet with the runs, about as frequently as when I had giardia. By the time I made it in the shala, my large intestine was clean and my bandhas were gone.

We take in the world with our five senses. We experience the sights, sounds, smells, tastes, and being touched by and touching the world. These signals refer back to the center of our being for processing. If an experience is not processed and released, it will get packed away and stored. The energy that is not released and not allowed to pass through is incomplete, unfinished. The stored unfinished energy is an impression. In Sanskrit, this is known as a samskara.

The thing is, our senses are often wrong. They are limited. Bats would laugh at our ability to hear, cats piss all over our ability to see, and that's only two examples of our limited senses. What we are interpreting is often all "in our head," and not what actually "is". I had two options when I was losing my crap, quite literally, before that first Led Intermediate practice with Sharath. As I saw it, I could call in sick and avoid going to this class for another week and face the shaming eyes of the boss on Monday, or I could move into the fear and process this experience. Process the diarrhea caused by fear, the fear of feeling unworthy of practicing with people who intimidated me. The inadequacy I felt from not being the cool kid in school repeated here again as an adult, alone in a foreign country. I didn't feel like the cool kid in school because I didn't have the cool toys that they had. In this case it was the cool asana that they were able to do with ease and a smile. What it came down to, was me comparing myself to others, and not comparing myself to who I was yesterday.

We get a few chances to process our experiences. If we choose to stuff our emotions, or eat them, then they may not come up again and we will face them in the next life. However, if it is our dharma this lifetime to overcome them, they will be regurgitated to be experienced all over again with more bitterness. Before we get to taste the experience again, it will ferment within us, undigested. So how do we work through digesting this experience? Let's start from the bottom and work our way up. We have established that we are moving out of pain and moving through Surya Namaskara A.

We are moving out of our past, whatever that had on us, and we are agreeing to process our unresolved energies, our samskaras. We have committed to moving into our version of health and happiness; whatever that looks like for ourselves that's not defined by a magazine or an Instagram photo.

With Surya B, we get right into expelling, evolving, and processing this journey. Surya B begins with a slight bend to the knees, ensuring that we are contracting the lower abdomen to lift up the chest, preventing it from collapsing. This movement activates the anal sphincter, if it hadn't been activated before. It ensures that what you have when you started this healing formula, on this journey, is not going to be leaking out but will be burned up.

The large intestine is responsible for retaining the necessary fluids from the food we have ingested and it's responsible for pushing out what we no longer need. When we step the right foot forward, we are squeezing the right side of the abdomen. The right side of the abdomen is the ascending part of the large intestine. This is the part where the small intestine meets the large intestine. Anatomically, we call this area the cecum. Placing physical pressure on the right side of the abdomen helps to move processed food from the small intestine along, faster up the large intestine. Contracting the right side can be thought of as wringing out a wet towel, squeezing beneficial fluids back into the blood stream. But to wring out a towel properly, we need to twist both ends, and that is why we subsequently put the left foot forward.

This squeezing and compression of the right side continues in Utthita Trikonasana, and even deeper in Utthita Parshvakasana. It is also why we place the right foot into Padmasana first, in Ardha Baddha Padmottasana. This "simple" procedure of placing the right foot at the sigmoid colon, the "S" shaped intersection of the colon to the large intestine, places physical pressure on the area, to lock the waste from moving back up, and it prevents diarrhea from 'leaking' out. Throughout the rest of the asana in the formula of a yoga practice that deals with digestion, this pressure and wringing out of the towel is going to continue to deepen. When practicing Triang Mukhaepada Paschimattasana in the sequence, we hold constant pressure on the ascending colon for five breaths while in the asana. This is like squeezing the towel and holding it. In the asanas that precede it, we are locking off or holding pressure on part of the intestine, but not completely closing down an entire side. In this asana, we express more of the good fluids back to the bloodstream for our benefit. While in the asana it is important to breathe slowly, making the experience count.

One of the most challenging digestive asana is Marichyasana D. Locking the hands can be demanding. There is tremendous pressure on the joints, shoulders, and the sacral-iliac joints and it seems impossible if there are knee or spine injuries.

If we stepped the left foot forward first in Surya B or the other asana, not only is it the 'incorrect method,' but we risk moving food from the colon, back into the large intestine (this is also an argument for why it is good practice to defecate BEFORE practicing). The colon is where food ferments and gets ready to leave. You just don't want that shit coming back. There isn't much separating the colon from the large intestine. To keep the shit from getting out, we have a strong sphincter muscle that holds it in the colon. But the only division between the colon and the large intestine is an 'S' shaped fold that keeps the fermenting waste product from moving back up to the intestine.))<>((

One thing to note with practicing twists like; Utthita Trikonasana, Parshvakasana, Mari C & D, there is excessive pressure being exerted on the large intestine. If the individual has a history of diverticulitis or has a colostomy\ileostomy, extra care must be taken when performing these asanas. They are still assessable to the practitioner, but they may need to be modified.

* Society for Neuroscience. "'Second brain' neurons keep colon moving: Brain in the gut coordinates activity of millions of neurons to propel waste through digestive system." ScienceDaily. ScienceDaily, 29 May 2018. <www.sciencedaily.com/releases/ 2018/05/180529132122.htm>.

One thing to think about is that with epigenetics (environmental factors that turn on expressions in genes), as we get older, we can get healthier; with +thinking and +diet. Diseases can be thought of as a test. Will we change our lifestyle?

HEART AND TONGUE

I didn't want to separate the organ systems into groups because I didn't want to give the impression that the systems work independently of each other. This seems like a, 'No shit Sherlock' moment, but I didn't realize this very basic concept until a Human Systems Development class in college. Until that point, I believed that the digestive system worked with food. Period. The respiratory system dealt with gas exchange, oxygen and carbon dioxide. Period. And the circulatory system dealt with blood. Period. I didn't recognize that the nutrients from the food we eat are carried around in the blood stream to their targets. Or that the organs, ALL of the organs, are made from the food that we eat. That all of the organs are supported by the blood that enriches them with oxygen and nutrients. I also didn't realize that the lungs needed the contractions of the heart muscle to bring the oxygen around the body in the blood. I thought these gasses floated around inside of us, like the broken down bits of food. As such they eventually would get to where they were going.

There was this big "Oh!" moment for me in that freshman class, followed by this bit of anger for being taught the systems independently and lead to believe otherwise. For this, and other reasons, I am not going to separate the Respiratory and Cardiovascular systems. I will attempt to put the pieces together in one category. Please understand though, that these systems are unified with the other systems to form the perfect being that you are.

"Your heart is one of the masterpieces of creation. It is a phenomenal instrument. It has the potential to create vibrations and harmonies that are far beyond the beauty of pianos, strings, or flutes. You can hear an instrument, but you feel your heart. And if you think that you feel an instrument, it's only because it touched your heart. Your heart is an instrument made of extremely subtle energy that few people come to appreciate." - The Untethered Soul Michael A. Singer

When you ask a three-year-old to point to themselves, they point to their chest. Most adults do this as well when talking about themselves. There is a reason that we point to the heart and not the head when talking about ourselves. The heart is the center. It's function is vital to the essence of who we are on our spiritual journey. You can be alive without brain wave activity, but when the heart stops it's sinus rhythm, so does our journey with this lifetime.

The heart is self-sustaining. That little guy doesn't need you to think about it doing its job. In fact, it's usually doing much better without our involvement. For instance, remember when you first walked into a yoga room and you see a few bodies contorted like a pretzel and there is this odd sound of breathing and silence in the room? Remember what it was like when you have to actually remember the asana the teacher taught you only five seconds ago? That panic, the fright, the thought's that arise, those are us interfering with the heart doing its job of chugging along at a steady pace, making sure you get to the end of your spiritual journey. The heart is one of those organs controlled by the autonomic nervous system. The autonomic nervous system is the part that runs automatically. It doesn't require cognitive thought. However, thought, along with emotions, things we see or hear, and a few other factors, do affect the heart rate via chemicals in the blood and neurotransmitters.

The neurotransmitters come from the brain via the autonomic nervous system. The autonomic nervous system is divided into two groups, the sympathetic, and parasympathetic. The sympathetic nervous system increases the heart rate by releasing epinephrine into the blood. The parasympathetic system slows the heart rate by releasing acetylcholine. Acetylcholine is released from the vagus nerve to slow down the heart rate. Comprised mostly of sensory nerve fibers, the vagus nerve relays information to the brain about how we feel. Parasympathetic nerve fibers in the vagus nerve are responsible for control of the heart, lungs, and the digestive track. It is also responsible for stopping peristalsis (digestion), sweating, and part of our speech. In the Su Wen, chapter 9 from the 2nd century BCE, it states that 'the heart opens to the tongue.' The heart governs our ability to choose words. Speak from the heart. Listen to what it has to say. Exercise this connection.

When we think of exercise, we commonly think of working out skeletal muscles and the heart muscle. The heart normally contracts 50 to 100 times in a minute when at rest. It receives a signal from the vagus nerve to contract, moving blood throughout the body, to provide oxygen and nutrients to the organs. If something disrupts this impulse, we can experience; Shortness Of Breath (SOB), lightheadedness, chest pain, fainting, or palpitations (an uncomfortable irregular sensation in the chest like "flopping"), A resting heart rate above 100 is a sign that the heart is not providing enough oxygen to the body, or that there is an electrical malfunction.

It is not uncommon for athletes and yogis to have a lower resting heart rate below 50 beats per minute. This is because, with their training, the parasympathetic functions of the vagus nerve are trained as well. If we concentrate our minds on breathing only, the state of an asana will be changed. On the other hand, if we concentrate only on an asana's state, our breathing will be irregular.

Our heart rate is directly linked to our breathing. When we inhale the heart rate increases. When we exhale the heart rate slows down. It does this in order to optimize oxygen uptake and carbon dioxide removal in the lungs.* With a smooth, long exhale, the circulatory system, lungs and heart, are telling the brain that we are safe. The optimized gas exchange in individuals who practice activities that slow the exhale rate, minimize the workload of the heart.**
Turtles breathe four times a minute and live for over 300 years. Indian philosophy has an idea that an individual's lifetime is predetermined by a set amount of breaths. With training, we can slow down our breathing and decrease our heart rate, extending our lives. "When, like the tortoise which withdraws its limbs on all sides, he (a sage) withdraws his senses from the sense-objects, then his wisdom becomes steady." -Bhagavad Gita II-58.

Pranayama can bring up a lot of fear. The sustained breath holding is similar to drowning. Or training for free diving. FEAR is a reaction to current events, things that are happening to our immediate person. It is common to be in a sympathetic overdrive these days with our anxious and excited lives. We often say that we are busy, and multitasking. Jobs, family, asana practice, fruit detox, coffee enema, our minds are all over the place. Far from the wise and steady tortoise. If we experience fear, stress, anxiety, illness, fever, or pain, the heart rate increases. It increases by stimulating the sympathetic system.

Fear and anxiety are different. Anxiety is a worry about a future event. Think like, anxiety is worrying about Kapotasana while having your morning coffee. Fear is actually doing the backbend with your teacher. OR, anxiety is thinking about an asthma attack and not having an inhaler, not being able to breathe, and sitting with your hands on your knees supporting your chest from collapsing. Fear, and the fear response, has been preserved throughout evolution because it ensures our survival by generating an appropriate behavioral response, fight or flight. The brain records fear, what caused it, what actions were taken; and will cause the individual to remember details surrounding the situation. With this recording, we are able to, sometimes forced to, re-live our fears. Hopefully, to have a finer tuned response the next time we encounter the stimuli. The only way around the recording that I know is to practice.

'Practice and all is coming' is a phrase that is terribly cliche. I have heard it as a way to pass over an answer and I understand others take comfort in that phrase. Practice and ALL is coming . . . I seldom hear, practice and stress is coming. Practice and fear is coming. But they come. And IF we talk about them, we only talk about them looking back in hindsight. We paint a pretty picture of how we overcame (insert asana name here) or we didn't let (insert situation) control us. But, practice and anxiety is coming.

Control your breathing grasshopper.

*Hayano J, Yasuma F, Okada A, Mukai S & Fujinami T (1996). Respiratory sinus arrhythmia. A phenomenon improving pulmonary gas exchange and circulatory efficiency. *Circulation* **94**, 842–847.
**Ben-Tal, A. , Shamailov, S. S. and Paton, J. F. (2012), Evaluating the physiological significance of respiratory sinus arrhythmia: looking beyond ventilation–perfusion efficiency. The Journal of Physiology, 590: 1989-2008. doi:10.1113/jphysiol.2011.222422

BREATHING

If we focus on only one aspect of the entire yoga practice, we fail. Just as the breath cannot be separated from the man, the mind cannot be separated either. The body, the breath, and the mind are linked. All aspects of our human existence are linked. We are here to serve. Serve each other.

If we practice yoga only for ourselves, only for an asana or for a 'good stretch', we will certainly fail to reach enlightenment. We will serve to separate ourselves from our fellow beings. We will separate ourselves from compassion, understanding, and empathy, making ourselves into a flexible asshole.

Flexible or not, all humans depend on breathing to live. Specifically, humans need oxygen for life. The air that we breathe is about 21% oxygen, even at the top of a mountain when it feels difficult to breathe, it's still about 21%. All of our cells require oxygen for metabolism, but the heart and brain are particularly sensitive to a lack of oxygen. A shortage of oxygen to these organs for a few minutes is fatal.

Oxygen is transported around the body in the blood attached like a magnet to an iron-containing protein called hemoglobin (Hgb). We breathe oxygen in through the nose, where those hairs and mucus filter out dirt and dust particles. The air swirls around in the back of the nose giving it time to warm up and humidify before traveling down the trachea. The trachea is about an inch in diameter with cartilage rings around it to prevent it from collapsing or over inflating. Like when you suck on a straw with a piece of boba or coconut flesh inside, these rings keep the shape of the trachea.

The trachea divides into branches called the bronchi, that further subdivide into the bronchiole. When the diaphragm contracts, air is pulled into the lungs and travels through these tubes that look like the roots of a tree. At the end of the bronchiole, are pods called alveoli that are continually fed blood from the heart. Alveoli is where gas exchange takes place in the lungs. The warm humidified air that we take in, swirls around inside these pods waiting to be carried through the body. If these pods are filled with smoke, or fluid, then we have less available area to release the waste and trade up for the oxygen that the body needs to function. Oxygen (O_2) is more attractive and fits together better with the magnetic force of the hemoglobin in the blood than carbon dioxide (CO_2). When blood is squeezed through the tiny vessels around the alveoli, CO_2 pops off and is replaced with O_2. The blood, now rich in O_2, travels back to the heart via the pulmonary vein, to the top left chamber of the heart.

The heart is the emperor controlling all the other organs, it is at our center and the root of our life. It is protected and held in place by the pericardium. Divided into 4 chambers, left and right, top and bottom, the heart is responsible for the flow of blood throughout the body, and is often thought of as the body's main energy center, the 4th chakra, our place of feeling.

"An energy center is an area within your being through which your energy focuses, distributes, and flows. This energy flow has been referred to as Shakti, Spirit, and Chi, and it plays an intricate part in your life. You feel the heart's energy all the time." The Untethered Soul - Michael Singer.

The heartbeat/energy flow can be felt physically, through palpating a person's pulse, and monitored electrically, through an EKG. Each contraction and relaxation is called a heartbeat. When the heart relaxes, blood moves through one way valves from the top areas of the heart (atrium) to the lower half called the ventricles. When it receives a signal from the vagus nerve, an electrical impulse contracts the muscles around the ventricles moving blood away from the heart. Blood pressure is a measurement of how strong the contraction is. The top number is the amount of force the heart is exerting to push blood around the body. The bottom number is the amount of pressure it takes to fill the heart back up with blood to do it all over again. The oxygen rich blood leaves the left ventricle to the aorta. The aorta is the largest artery in the body. Arteries are blood vessels with a muscular lining around the tube that produce a contraction, called a pulse that can be felt under certain parts of the body. The pulse is synchronized with the heartbeat to move blood rich in O2 further along the body and away from the heart.

Arteries divide, and branch out becoming smaller and smaller in diameter until the smooth muscle disappear. When the smooth muscle disappears, the diameter of the tube is only wide enough for a single cell to fit through at a time. These tiny tubes are called capillaries, where oxygen is exchanged for carbon dioxide, and sugars and other nutrients are picked up into, and exchanged in the bloodstream. As the blood cell moves through the tiny capillary, it must distort its shape, which changes the magnetic bond between the hemoglobin and oxygen and allows for the larger CO2 molecule to take its place for the return journey back to the heart. The capillaries eventually join back together, after covering the surface of a particular tissue, to form veins. Unlike arteries, veins have no muscles to move blood around the body and are reliant upon the structural muscles to facilitate the movement of blood. This is one of the reasons veins are sometimes visible protruding under the surface of the skin. Veins link up, growing larger in diameter, until emptying into two main branches called the inferior and superior venae cava. These branches almost continuously empty deoxygenated blood into the right atrium.

When the heart relaxes, the one way valve opens up allowing this blood to enter into the right ventricle. As before, when the heart receives an electrical signal to contract, the ventricles contract. The blood carrying CO2 moves away from the heart and to the lungs through the pulmonary artery. This artery, like the others, divide and spread out into capillaries around the alveoli of the lungs, the air pods. The blood cell is squeezed again, changing the shape of the hemoglobin and bumping out the CO2 for O2. When the diaphragm relaxes, it compresses the lungs pushing the carbon dioxide up and out of the body.

HOW TO IMPROVE THE BREATH

I didn't know what drowning was at two years old, but I knew I didn't like it. I grew up on, in, and above the water. My parents set off cruising in a sailboat when I was about 6 months old. In the first grade we took a sailboat through the Panama Canal. At 35 I bought a sailboat of my own and lived on it. I love the water. Even my birth sign is water. It also holds my most deep seated fear, drowning.

When I was about two, maybe three, my mom was playing with me at the beach and took me deeper than I could stand in the strong surf. A wave swept her off of her feet and she wasn't able to hold me and keep herself above the water. In that moment, she pushed me to the surface, but I couldn't swim. I remember the panicked look on her face distorted underwater. I remember not being able to breathe, seeing red, and then nothing. I don't remember what happened next or how I got to the beach, but I did, obviously, and I was quickly enrolled in swimming classes.

I took to the water like a fish. I spent time jumping off bridges into water, swimming to the bottom of the pool, holding my breath and swimming back and forth multiple lengths of the pool. My first 'real' job was swimming with sharks in the Bahamas, tagging them for behavioral research.

There is a sport called free-diving where the diver holds their breath and dives down to a depth, without the use of a breathing device like a scuba tank. The current depth record is 214m (702.1 feet) where Herbert Neitsch held his breath for 4 minutes and 24 seconds. Most of these athletes hold their breath for 9 to 11 minutes. Scientists are still a bit puzzled by the physiology of it. Physically, according to some calculations, at 30-40m the lungs would collapse, but we know that this isn't the case.

> "There is an element of physicality but it's mainly mental. That's what is incredible about free diving. It's not about your physical

ability, but about your mental skills and mental training basically. You need to let go of everything that you know and everything that makes you feel good or bad. And so it's a very liberating process. But equally you need to stay completely aware of your body and where you are, entirely in the moment." - Martina Amati

As the sport of free diving has evolved so has their training. These athletes use CO_2 and O_2 tables as a guide that pushes their body's tolerance of dealing with high CO_2 or low O_2. High levels of CO_2 in the blood are those STRONG burning feelings of needing to breathe. The feeling I felt as a kid drowning in the ocean.

There are a few apps you can download to improve your diving breath holds. I use Low2 and Eddie Stern's breathing app. They are not a substitute for a teacher. I will say that again. They are NOT a substitute for a pranayama teacher. However, they can give you a decent idea about pranayama, and you will be a better free diver from practicing. But how is holding your breath going to improve your health? That's the real question. Apps can be fun. Yoga practice can be fun. Heroin can be fun too. But are they contributing to your overall wellbeing? What is the point of holding your breath and being able to transport more oxygen in your blood?

In the event that a scuba diver surfaces too quickly without depressurizing his body to the change in atmosphere, they get a condition known as 'the bends.' Dissolved gas in the bloodstream come out of solution and form bubbles, that get stuck in joints, causing paralysis or even death. The method used to treat the bends, is to place the diver in Hyperbaric Oxygen Therapy. This involves breathing pure oxygen in a pressurized chamber or room. In those conditions, the lungs can take in more oxygen than at normal air pressure. In an oxygen rich environment, a substance in the body is released that stimulates the growth of living cells like stem cells, and the body can easily fight off infections. Some infections that are commonly treated with Hyperbaric O_2 Therapy are skin or bone infections, gangrene, diabetic ulcers, and there are claims that it can help with HIV, Asthma, Cancer, and Allergies. Because the cost of a hyperbaric chamber is about $5,000 to $35,000, and most of us don't have that laying around, we find alternatives to condition our bodies and improve our daily use of oxygen. Through a pranayama practice or dive training, the body is being conditioned over time to increase the available O2. The idea behind breath retention and improving the CO2 hold, is that the body makes better use of the available oxygen in the blood. Essentially we are squeezing every ounce out of the breath. Every ounce out of life.

Pranayama breathing is different from the type of breathing we do during the asana practice. There are some similarities where the breath is sometimes held to bind the hands or getting the foot behind the head. Note that this is not the correct method, although effective. In the case for asana practice and those difficult binds, the body is being physically restrained. The lungs are not able to expand to their full capacity when in the deep binds of the asana, and in those instances we are clearing parts of our lungs that do not get used in the normal breathing cycle outside of practice. Typically the lungs can hold 6L of air. In a normal breathing cycle, we only take in 3.5L keeping 2.3L in reserve.** When we are twisted in those 'fun' asana, the reserve volume physically changes and is being used because of the physical restraint on the body. Asana in effect cleans the reserve volume of our lungs ever day in practice, like brushing our teeth every day to prevent plaque and bacteria buildup.

* Aversa, Raffaella and Petrescu, Relly Victoria and Apicella, Antonio and Petrescu, Florian Ion, The Basic Elements of Life's (December 17, 2016). American Journal of Engineering and Applied Sciences, Volume 9, Issue 4, Pages 1189-1197, DOI : 10.3844/ajeassp.2016.1189.1197. Available at SSRN: https://ssrn.com/abstract=3074489

**https://en.wikipedia.org/wiki/Lung_volumes

AWAKENING TO THE HAPPINESS OF ONE'S SELF REVEALED

How many peripheral arteries are occluded in Marichyasana D? Who thinks about this stuff . . .? "Inhale," he tells me as he lifts my arm holding my wrist.
"Exhale." My arm is taken across the knee, down and around so that my fingers are touching the shin of the opposite foot which has disappeared inside my stomach.
"Teaching side," he says with a head bobble pulling the other arm around my back connecting my fingers together.
"Hold."
White knuckle grip, I try to keep my fingers from coming apart. I'm taking shallow breaths so that my stomach doesn't push the knee any further away. I've been sweating so much that at any moment the arm is going to slide off of the knee it is wrapped around.

I was in Miami, visiting my Pop's and practicing at the Miami Life Center with Tim. I had forgotten about the humidity and about how much sweat the human body can produce. I didn't have a towel to put over my knee to give me an extra edge of support. I was new to this practice, maybe 9 months in, I had no idea what he meant about 'teaching side.' Two months earlier, his wife Kino did a workshop at the studio I practiced at in Chicago. She was talking about how asana is supposed to be a comfortable seat. That is the rough translation from Sanskrit to English. "Can you imagine drinking a cup of tea in Marichyasana D," she asked us during a discussion on twists. We are supposed to be that comfortable. That got a lot of laughs. My BS radar went up then, with lights and sirens screaming, 'Easy for her to say!'. How is one supposed to find 'comfort' in Marichyasana D with a heel digging into the gut, a knee in the chest, a head craned looking backwards like the Exorcist, and little fingers grasping to hold this shape together.

I filed this tea drinking BS, in my wacky Mysore hocus pocus woo woo folder for a few years. Every couple of weeks this tea idea would haunt me in Marichyasana D, maybe that's why I needed to urinate before this asana? After some time, like years, I no longer needed assistance getting into this asana. D didn't require towels to dry sweat, evacuation of the bowels before practice or a minimum of 10+ hours of fasting before attempting it wasn't necessary. At this point years later, there was a different asana that was consuming those thoughts and actions. I forgot about the tea.

In 2010 I fractured and dislocated the left clavicle during a 4th of July party that involved a kiddie pool. Six weeks of modified practice without any weight or pressure on the shoulder, meant that I had to relearn the entire primary series again. I was super trepidatious attempting Marichyasana D again, or any of the Marichyasana.

Do you know why 'they' recommend consulting a MD before beginning an exercise routine?

The skinny of it is that if you have a blood clot or a piece of plaque (fat, cholesterol, and calcium) in your veins and it becomes dislodged and makes its way back to the heart it could get lodged in a smaller blood vessel blocking the blood flow and cause a heart attack or stroke. If one of these clots gets stuck in the lungs it could cause shortness of breath, chest pain, or the coughing up of blood. This is called a pulmonary embolism. That's a very simple explanation, but you understand that it's a bad thing.

The same, 'they' recommend getting up and walking around on an airplane while traveling for long periods: so that the blood doesn't pool and clot, or dislodge one of these plaque formations, sending it back to the heart.

Conventional health care is fundamentally concerned with the prevention and alleviation of suffering. The responsibility for the alleviation or prevention of that suffering is rarely discussed,* and who is responsible? I believe that we are responsible for our health. We, being the individual, along with MD's, RN's, Pharmacists, Acupuncturists, insurance companies, hospitals, parents, and politicians. The responsibility cannot be pawned off to someone else. The Mayo Clinic recommends getting 30 min of moderate activity most days of the week to prevent cardiovascular disease. It's not the politicians responsibility to ensure that I got in my 30 minutes of activity, it's mine. But it is the politician's responsibility to ensure that EVERYONE has access to health care. So, I dragged myself into the changing room and took care of my health. In time I learned how to come up from backbends without blacking out. I learned how to breathe correctly and made the heart happy.

Practicing Yoga makes the individual strong from the inside by improving the organ systems. It allows the individual to become responsible for their own health and develop a responsibility for it. Understanding our individual responsibility to our health and health care prevents the unnecessary suffering of others. Most athletes don't worry about clots, also known as DVT's (deep vein thrombosis) because they are young and healthy. Blood clots usually affect older unhealthy individuals, but can affect everyone, and Nurse Morgan knows that a bone fracture increases your risk of developing a DVT and I fractured the clavicle. My mind was not still in practice. I was afraid of a DVT and afraid of dislocating the clavicle again. That's when the question that started this entire search for a scientific meaning behind the practice began. How many peripheral arteries are occluded in Marichyasana D?

The answer has awakened an internal happiness for me. I began researching what Jois said about the asana. I read other blogs, books, watched videos and never found a satisfactory answer. I had so many questions, I still have so many questions. What, if any, are some scientific and medical explanations for the benefits of doing asana? I know there are benefits, but give me the science.

There are 18 major peripheral arteries in the body, 9 on each side. In the neck, arms, and legs. Arteries are like mini hearts; they push blood further along in the body bringing oxygen and nutrients to that area of the body. In Marichyasana D we occlude 12 of them.

The volume of blood inside the body during our asana practice does not change. When we place significant pressure on the arterial wall restricting the free flow of blood to the region of the body supplied by that artery, we build up the blood volume to the area before the artery. With restricted blood flow to the peripheral limbs, when we are in the state of the asana breathing for 5 breaths, the heart receives a higher volume of blood which also registers a higher concentration of CO_2. To compensate for the change in the body's pH from a buildup of CO_2 and the increased blood volume, the heart rate, and respiratory rate increase. Meaning, we breathe faster and shallower to circulate more blood through the heart. With a daily practice, over the course of time, our breathing will begin to slow down as each breath is able to receive more O_2 and expel more CO_2. Essentially, the breath becomes more efficient. The muscles of the arteries also begin to strengthen which means that it allows for the movement of this larger volume of blood.* This means that the vasculature of an athlete is more open. This is why physicians do not think to look for DVT's in athletes. Think hot dog down a hallway.

After 5 breaths in Marichyasana D, the increased volume that the heart has adjusted to, suddenly drops as the arteries are no longer occluded. Blood, rich with oxygen, rushes to fill the starved tissue in the feet and hands, legs and arms.

Ever stand up too quickly and felt dizzy or lightheaded? Maybe you were dehydrated, or sick, on medication, or your blood sugar was low when this happened? That lightheaded feeling is the brain not getting enough blood. The volume of blood in the arteries was not enough to adequately supply the brain with oxygen. This results in a sudden loss of blood pressure, and the vasovagal responses to black out to re-direct blood to vital organs. When we transition between asanas we are decreasing the pressure in the arteries and veins. This happens quickly, usually in one breath; we go from contraction to expansion. It takes extra work for the entire circulatory system to keep up with the change. More work than simple cardiovascular exercise. Yoga is cardiovascular exercise if the heart rate stays elevated typically for more than 30 minutes. The flowing between asana also conditions the arteries and veins to expand and contract with constant changing volumes. If the veins and arteries don't keep up, we black out.

*Shepherd, Lois L., Rethinking Health Law: Assuming Responsibility. Wake Forest Law Review, Forthcoming; FSU College of Law, Public Law Research Paper No. 189. Available at SSRN: https://ssrn.com/abstract=882477

**Vascular adaptation in athletes: is there an 'athlete's artery'? Daniel J. Green Angela Spence Nicola Rowley Dick H. J. Thijssen Louise H. Naylor
First published: 28 March 2012 https://doi.org/10.1113/expphysiol.2011.058826

REPRODUCTIVE SYSTEM

Can yoga improve the health of the human reproductive system? Should women practice yoga during their cycle? How does yoga help with regulating the menstrual cycle?

Our current testing standards do not have a way to quantify or qualify Traditional Chinese Medicine (TCM) or Ayurveda, but if there was not any validity behind them, their practice would have disappeared long ago. Current western treatments are relatively new compared to TCM and Ayurvedic treatments. Western treatments are focused on making a patient feel better for a while by treating their symptoms, but the underlying cause of the symptoms is not fully addressed. There is a push in the conventional medical community to treat the root of the symptoms, and consequently there is a progression towards TCM and other natural remedies as evidenced by The World Health Organization (WHO) accepting TCM into the fold.

Not everyone is welcoming of natural remedies. In an open letter to WHO, Scientific American wrote; To include TCM in the *ICD* is an egregious lapse in evidence-based thinking and practice. Data supporting the effectiveness of most traditional remedies are scant, at best.* Most acupuncture studies do not meet current testing standards because TCM focuses on the individual and not the symptom. Both systems are in agreement that the individual is not the symptom, but we cannot quantify an individual separate from the symptom with our current testing model. Research into TCM has found unique structures at acupuncture points and acupuncture channels using MRI (magnetic resonance imaging), infrared imaging, LCD thermal photography, ultrasound and other CT imaging methods, and have named these structures the 'primo-vascular system.** While this is not direct and enough evidence to support the claims of TCM and Ayurveda about channel theory and nadis being accepted into medical practices, there is significant progress into acceptance.

So how do we quantify claims that certain asana and the practice of yoga can benefit the reproductive system?

There are many tools in our toolbox to treat our health. We want the 'best' tool to get the job done. One question we need to be asking ourselves is, "Is this tool duct tape?" "Being skeptical can be good. Critical thinking can be good, but take it too far and it can turn into cynicism…" - *The Miracle Equation*, Hal Elrod. Our knowledge of science is evolving. What we know to be true today, scientists are hard at work disproving.

An open cadaver on an autopsy table will show the organs, soft tissues, bones, nerves, blood vessels, etc. Nowhere inside can we see emotions. There is no fear, love, joy, loneliness, or happiness that can be seen with our eyes. Scientists have disproved that emotions exist only in our heads. Emotions can be measured.*** Simply because we can't see it with our eyes, doesn't mean that it doesn't exist. Our senses only perceive a limited view. It's comical that, based on this, we think we have it all figured out.

In May of 2019 the World Health Organization (WHO) included Acupuncture and Traditional Chinese Medicine remedies into the 11th version of the *International Statistical Classification of Diseases and Related Health Problems* (ICD-11). Documentation of TCM medical practices dates to 1766 BCE where healers use various parts of plants and animals to treat patients. Traditional Chinese Medicine is based on the concept of Qi, a system of energy that flows along meridians in the body to maintain health.**

From India, The Varaha Upanishad (13-16 BCE) describes nadis as a pathway that 'penetrates the body from the soles of the feet to the crown of the head. In them is prana, the breath of life and in that life abides,' (VU 54).

It's impossible to deny that there is a flow of energy through the body. "It's been called by many names. In ancient Chinese medicine, it is called Qi. In yoga, it is called Shakti. In the West, it is called Spirit….the yogis call energy centers chakras." - *The Untethered Soul*, Michael A. Singer. Traditional Oriental Medicine links these centers with our internal organs.

Both systems involve using natural remedies to allow the body to heal itself.

The path of yoga is a natural remedy that works on the individual's energies. The sequence of asana or postures, work together in a series that progressively restores health to an individual. "If one first practices the Surya Namaskara and then the other asanas, then one's blood will become hot and pure, and will flow to every part of the body." - *The Yoga Mala*, Jois)

The dynamic movements of Surya Namaskara's begins by heating up the blood and moving the nutrients (Prana/Qi) to all parts of the body. The standing sequence that follows, uses the energy and heat created to build a healthy digestive system.

In Maslow's Hierarchy of needs, food, warmth, and safety are the basic needs that must be met, before an individual can focus on psychological needs including reproduction and intimate relationships. After addressing the basic needs, eventually the individual can turn their focus to self-fulfillment goals, including creative activities.

Similarly, the sequence of a yoga practice works to first establish warmth and safety in the individual and then improve their digestion through the practice of standing asanas. The benefits of each of these standing asana are to restore digestive health and stabilize the spinal column. Beginning with Utthita Hasta Padangushtasana, the benefits continue to focus on digestion and the resolution of pre-existing conditions but introduce a new benefit; to the hip joints and areas of reproduction. Interestingly this asana and the one that follows, Ardha Baddha Padmottanasana, have the first two fingers encircling the great toe.

In TCM theory, at the great toe are the entry points to the Foot Tai Yin and Foot Jue Yin channels on the medial and lateral side of the nail respectively. The Foot Tai Yin point, Yin Bái (Sp1) regulates the blood and can be used to treat menorrhagia and uterine bleeding. The Foot Jue Yin entry point, Dà Dūn (Lv1) also helps with regulating menstruation. Ardha Baddha Padmottanasana further helps to regulate the menstrual cycles, by invigorating the Ren Mai and Chong Mai when the lateral malleolus places pressure on the proximal end of the thigh on the lateral border of the abductor longs muscle. This point is known as Yin Lián (Lv 11). These asanas benefit everyone who practice them.

* https://www.scientificamerican.com/article/the-world-health-organization-gives-the-nod-to-traditional-chinese-medicine-bad-idea/
** https://www.healthcmi.com/Acupuncture-Continuing-Education-News/1230-new-ct-scans-reveal-acupuncture-points
*** https://www.ncbi.nlm.nih.gov/pmc/articles/PMC5298234/

REPRODUCTIVE QI

"In every culture and in every medical tradition before ours, healing was accomplished by moving energy." – Albert Szent-Gyorgyi, Biochemist / Nobel Prize Winner.

The practice of Yoga, Tai-Chi, Qi Gong, and the practice of TCM are energy practices.
According to TCM there are 14 channels that originate from the Chong Mai. In Ayurveda, the Chong Mai is named the Sushumna Nadi. From the Chong Mai, two channels branch from the Chong Mai and are known as the Ren Mai and Du Mai, or the Ida and Pingala respectively in Ayurveda. These channels are at the core of our body's development and the root of our essence.

In TCM the outer layers or channels deal with the lower levels of Maslow's Hierarchy of needs, and the chakras related to digestion. While the inner channels protect the heart and the essence of our beings. As the layers descend, we focus on higher level needs including reproduction. In order for these deeper layers to be addressed, we must make sure that the individual is healthy enough to reproduce. Scientifically, across the board, this is known as survival of the fittest, Darwin's theory of evolution.

For reproduction to take place, the individual needs to be physically and emotionally healthy. There are several contributing factors that lead to impotency; however, they all fall under two main categories; poor digestive health, and emotional health.

DIGESTIVE HEALTH
When a body is in poor health, it is unable to digest nutrients properly. Without proper nutrients the body goes into self-preservation mode. The body works to establish the lower levels of Maslow's needs. Reproduction is not a necessary function for survival.

If the body is receiving enough nutrients but not the proper ones to thrive, it will still operate on survival mode. Sex hormones are transported throughout the body in cholesterol. On a low cholesterol diet, hormones that control ovulation, and the production of semen are unable to reach their target organ, the ovaries and gonads. If someone has excessive levels of LDL cholesterol, this can reduce blood supply to these organs by blocking arteries and veins. This can also lead to a taxation on the liver as it needs to produce more bile to breakdown complex fat molecules for absorption and assimilation into the body.

Abstaining from sex, is a traditional Yogic practice, brahmacharya. Like fasting, it can be a valuable tool for cleansing and for learning about one's self. However, the tool can be misused. Each individual is different in their level of sexual need. Fasting from food or sex should never be forced upon an individual, and should arise from the individual's own feelings of a need for self-discipline. On the opposite end of the spectrum, excessive sex can drain the individuals reserve energy.

Another physical taxation on the body's ability for reproduction is lower back pain. Chronic lower back pain affects the functions of the kidneys and the Foot Jue Yin organ. The kidneys are physically located in the lower back and a portion of the Foot Jue Yin channel passes by the surface there. Chronic kidney disease causes menstrual irregularities, amenorrhea, and can lead to infertility.**** It is important to exercise and stretch this area to avoid lower back pain, sexual and reproductive problems.

EMOTIONAL HEALTH
Factors that contribute to poor emotional health around impotency, relate to our individual circumstances in life. When two people engaged in a sexual relationship are unresponsive or unable to have a level of openness about their expectations, insecurities and fears, a level of dissatisfaction is inevitable.

Men often feel pressured to preform or act in a certain way during intercourse. This often results in prematurely ejaculating without conscious control. Men who often fantasize about sex, can build up semen faster, causing them to ejaculate earlier during intercourse. In women, vaginal infections and menstrual cramps can be an expression of emotional stress and pressure. The inability of a women to orgasm, can sometimes be attributed to stress and pressure. In both of these instances, for men and women, feelings of; guilt, self-doubt, and fear can be linked back to their Foot Shao Yin organ. This is the organ that houses our essence and is the original fire.

In the case of bramacharya, when strict morals that do not originate from one's own desire for self-discipline, are forced upon an them, this can result in repressed anger. Anger that is pushed down and held inside affects the Foot Jue Yin organ and it's functions in reproduction by stagnating Qi.

Through the practice of yoga, an individual's digestive health can improve by following the sequence. As a result of following a specific sequence the individual often adapts a diet that includes foods that are pure, clean, conscious, and energy-containing, to assist the body in the development of their practice. As the individuals health improves their physical asana practice also improves allowing them to move beyond self-survival mode and into Maslow's next level of self-fulfillment needs, reproduction.

**** https://www.medscape.com/answers/238798-105290/how-does-chronic-kidney-disease-ckd-affect-reproductive-organs-and-fertility

THE FEMALE CYCLE

The major player in human reproduction is the Female. Unfortunately, because sexual health is taboo and not openly discussed, in part due to a patriarchal society, the waters around the female reproductive system are often murky.

Should women practice yoga, including inversions during their cycle? How does yoga help with regulating the menstrual cycle? Aside from acknowledging that some women have abdominal pain during menstruation, the topic of menstruation is not discussed in The Yoga Mala and is often avoided in yoga texts. 'A lot of women with strong Ashtanga practices at some point lose their periods, often due to a combination of low body weight and intense exercise," -Alison DeMaio, MD OB/GYN. This is common for high intensity sports across the board, known as athletic amenorrhea. Recent studies have highlighted that women with recreational exercise routines have a high prevalence of menstrual disturbances, with up to half of them having subtle or severe menstrual disturbances. Women with athletic amenorrhea often face persistent metabolic challenges in the form of intermittent or chronic energy imbalance due to increased energy expenditure or insufficient caloric intake.***** This can lead to osteoporosis, and other metabolic disorders. An excess of any yoga practice as a form of exercise, can lead to amenorrhea and a caution should be noted to all students of yoga.

It should be iterated here that yoga is medicine. As medicine, it needs to be respected. The asana is a meditation on the body and space. Pranayama is a meditation on the breath. If we only sit in the body and practice asana, we will get stuck in that layer, leading to disorders of the body. Pranayama uses the asana practice to be able to sit in comfort for extended periods of time. Meditation comes the combination of these skills.

"Some women find practice during their periods very helpful, and take rest the days following their cycle. After the shedding of the uterine lining, Progesterone sharply decreases and the drive, or energy, is decreased causing a need for rest. Endorphins released during practice help to counteract the decline in energy and mood allowing the individual to feel better." - Alison DeMaio, MD OB/GYN. On days 1-4[a] of menstruation, a gentle and modified form of practice can be done. There are some benefits of practice that can help with uterine contractions that help to descend and remove menstrual blood. The practitioner should focus on breathing and omit any inversions. Days 5-11, energy is beginning to build and levels of estrogen rise. With the gradual increase in estrogen, willpower and self-confidence rise. This can be a strong and dynamic time for the practice. Days 12-16, levels of estrogen drop and levels of progesterone rise. The rise in progesterone is to maintain a pregnancy if a viable egg is fertilized. Unlike estrogen which has a positive effect on the nervous system by stimulating an increase in serotonin, medium levels of progesterone have a depressing effect as they are metabolized by the liver and kidney. There is evidence to show that metabolized progesterone attaches to the GABA-A receptors preventing an uptake in serotonin, causing depressive feelings, or PMS.***** Higher levels of progesterone associated with pregnancy do not have this effect. From day 16-28, if an egg has not been fertilized there can be a gradual decrease in energy and a heightened feeling of sensitivity related to the metabolism of progesterone.

A particularly helpful asana for the regulation of menses and the symptoms of PMS, is Baddha Konasana. Looking at only 3 of the many points that are stimulated during the practice of this asana:

Gōng Sūn (Sp 4) Regulates the Chong Mai, the Sea of blood

Zhì Yīn (UB 67) Regulates pregnancy and childbirth (difficult labor)

Zú Lín Qì (GB 41) Distending pain of the breast, irregular menstruation, headaches

It is clear that practicing this asana alone can be beneficial to many women. One should be cautioned that practicing this asana alone, the blood is not warm and moving. In this case, the points are stimulated but there is no direction given to them where to go. Without direction they may or may not relay the message, and healing is not guaranteed.

In the Ashtanga Yoga primary series this asana is followed by Upavishta Konasana, Supta Konasana, Supta Padangushtasana, and Ubhaya Padangushtasana, four asanas that have the fingers wrapping around the big toe, the entry points to the Foot Tai Yin and Foot Jue Yin channels; points that regulate the blood and menstruation. These asanas are practiced well into the series when the blood is warm and moving freely. The message that was relayed in the practice of Buddha Konasana by stimulating those points now has a map, movement, and directions.

There is often 'the vague teaching of keeping the anus tight at all times which is a disservice to many women. My experience is that "anus" means a lot of things to a woman depending on the muscle use patterns and emotional conditioning. Sometimes they contract the glutes chronically. Sometimes only the urethra. Sometimes the obdurate externis.' -Angela Jamison, Ayurvedic practitioner and Certified Ashtanga Teacher. The cuing to 'keep the anus tight' and the often misunderstanding of the instruction, compounded by the surge of yoga teacher trainings in recent years due to the popularity of yoga in the west, is caused to believe that there is a link in the increase of blood clots during menses. Blood clots found in menstrual blood are usually formed in the vagina from heavy flow that collects inside the vagina long enough to clot. TCM refers to this as blood stasis.

There are no statistics, at the time of writing this, on how many women experience blood clots with their cycle. According to the mayo clinic, passing blood clots during a menstrual cycle is normal. Because it is 'normal' there are no studies done on how many women actually have this occurrence. While passing a nominal amount of blood clots, it is not dangerous and no immediate harm will arise.

According to TCM, it is a sign that there is something not quite right, and the body is no longer in harmony.

During days 1-4 of the cycle, practicing inversions is contraindicated for women unfamiliar with how their bodies respond to the practice. The primary concern with practicing these asanas during the cycle is back flow of menstrual blood. "Backflow is one of the theories of how endometriosis is formed, which is why it gets a lot of attention. When the uterus contracts as part of a normal menstrual cycle, some of the blood/endometrial tissue can travel via the tubes to the peritoneal cavity. We see this very often when we do laparoscopy on women during their period. You can see the blood down in the pelvis." - Alison DeMaio, MD OB/GYN.

Endometriosis is a condition where cells resembling the uterine lining, which is shed during menstruation, begin to grow outside the uterus. These lesions can cause excruciating pain, and in some cases, infertility. Typically, menstrual blood is pushed out through contractions of the uterus, not via gravity. Although the blood can be reabsorbed in the peritoneal cavity, there is no benefit in forcing the body to do this with inversions and risk a serious complication. An alternative to inversions can be, to lay with the legs up a wall, allowing the blood that is circulated in the lower limbs during practice to return to the system.

***** https://www.ncbi.nlm.nih.gov/pmc/articles/PMC2941235/#R2
****** http://www.medref.se/pms/backstrom_13.pdf
[a] Days are an approximation the average length of female menstruation is 28-29 days; however it is extremely variable.

CLOSING ASANA

The closing asana, mainly Baddha Padmasana, and Padmasana, should be performed by everyone. The benefits of Baddha Padmasana purify the Liver and Spleen. One should note that, the organs listed are not the western organs, but the organs associated with TCM.

In Baddha Padmasana the first two fingers once again wrap around the big toe, the entry points to the Foot Tai Yin and Foot Jue Yin channels, the point that regulates the blood and menstruation. In TCM, the Foot Tai Yin channel is often associated with the functions of the spleen/pancreas, and the Foot Jue Yin channel is associated with the liver.

When the individual takes Padmasana position crossing the legs on top of each other, two other main points are also stimulated. The Foot Shao Yang point Xuān Zhōng (GB 39), which is located about 3" above the external malleolus, on the anterior border of the fibula is the meeting point for all three Yang Foot Channels. This point clears excess heat and increases a connection to the Foot Shao Yin organ, the organ associated with the body's essence. Xuān Zhōng (GB 39) is stimulated when the left leg (associated with Yang energy) is crossed over the right leg (Yin energy) at Sān Yīn Jiāo (Sp 6). Sān Yīn Jiāo is located approximately 3" above the tip of the medial malleolus, posterior to the medial border of the tibia. It is the intersecting point of the three Yin Foot Channels and tonifies blood, regulates menstruation, treats impotence, headaches, insomnia, and dizziness.

There are many other points that are stimulated in preforming these two asanas, but the ones listed above are the main ones typically focused on and used in TCM treatments.
The evidence that practicing the Ashtanga Yoga primary series is beneficial to both men and women is overwhelming. The primary series formula restores and maintains health to the individual who

takes this practice. The individual who practices Ashtanga Yoga, must remember that they are taking medicine with each practice, powerful medicine that affects the body's energy. The sequence is designed in a way that promotes healing. Any variation from the sequence changes the prescription, and thus changes the benefits and desired outcome.

The doctor of the future will give no medicine, but will interest his patient in the care of the human frame, in diet and in the cause and prevention of disease. - Thomas Edison

It was my hope in writing this book that it begins a conversation into how yoga can be used as medicine. I am fortunate to have studied both oriental and conventional styles of medicine and recognize that I am not an expert in either field, however I have a unique understanding into how yoga benefits the human body because I have studied both of these medicines. The information I provided is intended to plant a seed so that you, the reader, will look further into an idea that resonates with you and dig deeper. I recognize that I only scratched the surface and this is not an exhaustive look into how healing and effective this medicine is. I am happy to share with you what I have learned.

Made in the USA
Middletown, DE
11 January 2022

58472661R00040